I0510270

LIVER DETOXIFICATION

*Step by step instructions to cleanse
Your Liver Naturally, Switch
Diabetes and High Blood Pressure*

Dr. Drake Robert

Table of Contents

CHAPTER ONE

The Liver

The liver is the biggest inside organ in the body, so it's protected to state we have to take great consideration of it. This football-sized organ is situated in the upper right piece of the stomach area.

What does the liver do?

The liver has numerous obligations and capacities in the body. This delightful organ couldn't be to a greater degree some assistance for those late evenings out drinking or the over-utilization of shoddy nourishment on a cheat day.

• The liver has an influence in the metabolic procedure of separating proteins and fats for storage.

• The purpose of this stockpiling is to in the long run convert it into the vitality we have to get past our everyday undertakings.

• Another enormous job the liver plays in the body is detoxification.

How does the liver dispose of poisons?

From medications and liquor to obscure outside substances, the liver helps channel and detoxify the materials not intended to be in our body. Guaranteeing poisons are securely expelled from your blood is one of the liver's most basic occupations.

• The initial step utilizes compounds and oxygen to

consume poisons, particularly greasy ones.

• The second detox step joins poisons with amino acids so they can be expelled from the liver through bile or pee.

• Specific outer poisons: certain prescriptions, nourishment added substances, additives, nourishment colorings, sugars, season enhancers, synthetics utilized in agribusiness, alcohols, unpredictable natural mixes, vapor, air contamination and numerous different variables.

By what means can compounds utilization help the detoxification procedure?

We need compounds in our bodies so as to do key jobs, for example, assimilation and detoxification. Numerous prohibitive weight control plans that individuals use today are deficient with regards to important chemicals.

We can help our admission of catalysts through numerous sorts of nourishments:

- Bananas

- Avocados

- Papaya

- Kefir

- Pineapple

- Miso

- Tempeh

- Soy sauce

- Sauerkraut

We can likewise expand our stomach related detoxification through teas and dietary enhancements.

• Purify™: The regular fixings in this vegan supplement bolsters solid separate and detoxification in the liver.

• Purify™ Complete Body Cleanse: There are 20 parcels for 10 days. This 10-day wash down offers an "entire body" way to deal with normal purging and detoxification. This recipe helps the body in the means expected to dispose of the poisons discharged into our bodies.

• These cases help the body's normal detoxification process by serving to both catch and dispose of undesirable poisons and other material.

• Green Tea: Catechins (cell reinforcements) from green tea increment the movement of pepsin (stomach related compound), the stomach related chemical that separates proteins in the stomach.

• Chai Tea: Cinnamon may help mitigate an assortment of stomach related sicknesses, for example, incidental gas, acid reflux, indigestion, stomach issues and queasiness.

• Kombucha Tea: This aged drink contains probiotics and compounds that help with absorption and liver detoxification.

In spite of the fact that the liver is answerable for detoxification, there are numerous things we can do to help further detoxify our bodies. Wellbeing and what we put in our bodies goes connected at the hip. It isn't unprecedented today for individuals to take radical fasting measures to detox their bodies and shed pounds. This system takes into consideration the best possible detoxification and disposal of lethal mixes."

For what reason is it imperative to purify and detoxify our liver?

The liver isn't your normal inward organ. More than some other organ, the liver empowers us to profit by the nourishment we eat. As the Crystal Star wellbeing online journal puts it, "without the liver... the change of nourishment into living vitality is nonexistent." Consuming poisons from our nourishment and beverages will cause a long haul impact on our liver that can be diminished. There are additionally parts of our everyday living that we can change or abstain from doing to keep our liver solid.

•	Avoiding liquor is extremely gainful for your liver, however we as a whole know it's not the least demanding when you go out or simply need a little wine with supper. Moderate utilization is alright!

•	Some medications and drugs may not be the least demanding for the liver to breakdown. It will consistently profit you to be mindful of what you might be taking and make certain to peruse the name.

• Flush it out! Water is something individuals today regularly don't drink enough of, and including lemon makes it far better. "Lemon and all citrus natural products contain nutrient C and minerals that lift substantial capacities and upgrade the purifying procedure, clearing out squanders. Flushing your liver resembles giving your body a decent pre-wash so your blood remains at ideal pH levels."

• Eating solid starches, fats, and proteins. As I said before, the liver is liable for the separating proteins and fats, so why not make the activity simpler? The nourishments recorded above are extraordinary for the liver just as almonds, coconut, pecans, chia, sunflower seeds, olives, and avocado.

CHAPTER TWO

Advantages of Cleansing

Concentrating on your wellbeing, body and psyche ought to be a main need. Detoxifying can prompt numerous positive upgrades, for example, an expansion in vitality levels. We as a whole have those days where we simply feel lethargic and unmotivated. Drinking a lot of water and devouring the correct nourishments can help increment your day by day vitality. Another approach to this is to know about lacks we may have and give our bodies the correct nutrients and minerals. Catalyst Nutrition™ Multi-nutrient is an astonishing framework of nutrients that upgrade every day vitality and give cancer prevention agents. These cancer prevention agents additionally help with boosting the invulnerable framework. Detoxifying the assortment of intruders may diminish the measure of colds you get a year. It is never past the point where it is possible to start detoxifying your body. The bioaccumulation of poisons increments as we get more established. Despite the fact that we as a whole wish detoxing would shield us from maturing, regardless we have to deal with our liver and different organs by keeping up sound propensities.

Could a Detox or Cleanse Help Your Liver?

You need to do all that you can to play a functioning job in your wellbeing. However, in the event that you think you need a liver detox (otherwise called a liver rinse or flush), you should know there isn't a lot of it can accomplish for you.

Your liver is perhaps the biggest organ in your body. It assists expel with squandering items and procedures different supplements and meds. A great many people think a purify will enable their liver to expel poisons better after an excessive amount of liquor or undesirable nourishments. Some expectation it will enable their liver to work better every day. Many accept it'll help treat liver malady.

Like most detox techniques, a liver purify has explicit steps. You may need to quick or to just drink juices or different fluids for a few days. You may need to eat a confined eating regimen, or take home grown or dietary enhancements. Some detoxes likewise brief you to purchase an assortment of other business items. A few approaches may join a few of these strategies.

Is There Any Proof That Liver Detox Works?

There isn't any logical evidence that rinses evacuate poisons or make you more advantageous. The explanation detox diets may make you feel better is that they normally don't enable you to eat profoundly prepared nourishments. These nourishments contain strong fats and handled sugar. They're high in calories yet low in nourishment. Detox diets can likewise remove nourishments that you may be unfavorably susceptible or delicate to, similar to dairy, gluten, eggs, or peanuts.

Specialists state liver detoxes aren't significant for your wellbeing or how well your liver functions. There's no proof they help dispose of poisons after you've had an excessive amount of nourishment or liquor. There's additionally no proof that they fix liver harm that has just occurred.

Does Milk Thistle Help Your Liver?

Milk thorn is a herb that contains a compound called silybin. You may have heard that it enables your liver work to better and can help treat liver ailment. However, similarly as there isn't sufficient proof that liver detoxes work, there isn't sufficient to show that milk thorn or concentrates from it make your liver more advantageous.

There is some verification that mixes from milk thorn have improved the manifestations of specific sorts of liver infection. In any case, no examinations show that it treats the ailment itself.

Are Liver Detoxes Safe?

There are medicinal medications for different liver infections. In any case, nothing shows that detox projects or enhancements can fix liver harm. Truth be told, detoxes can hurt your liver. There are additionally things you have to think about these projects and items:

• Some organizations use fixings that could be hurtful. Others have made false claims about how well they treat genuine sicknesses.

• Unpasteurized juices can make you debilitated, particularly in case you're more established or have a debilitated invulnerable framework.

• If you have kidney ailment, a wash down that incorporates a lot of juice can exacerbate your ailment.

• If you have diabetes, make certain to check with your PCP before you consider any eating regimen that changes how you regularly eat.

• If you have to quick as a feature of a detox program, you can feel powerless, black out, have cerebral pains, or get dried out. On the off chance that you have hepatitis B that has caused liver harm, fasting can exacerbate the harm.

The most effective method to Keep Your Liver Healthy

Your general wellbeing and your qualities influence your liver. Diet do as well, way of life, and condition. There are straightforward, rational advances you can take to help keep your liver sound without uncommon detox programs. These rules can be particularly significant on the off chance that you have certain things that make liver infection more probable, similar to overwhelming liquor use or a family ancestry of liver sickness. You should:

• Limit the measure of liquor you drink. Converse with your PCP about what's ideal for you.

• Eat a well-adjusted eating regimen consistently. That is 5-9 servings of foods grown from the ground, alongside fiber from vegetables, nuts, seeds, and entire grains. Additionally, make certain to incorporate protein to help chemicals that help your body detox normally.

• Keep a sound weight, or shed pounds in the event that you have to.

• Exercise consistently in the event that you can. Check with your PCP in the event that you haven't been dynamic.

• Cut down on hazardous conduct that can prompt viral hepatitis:

- Avoid illicit medications, however on the off chance that

you do utilize them,
don't share needles or
straws to infuse or
grunt them.

o   Don't   share   razors,
toothbrushes, or other family unit
articles.

o   Only get tattoos from a
sterile shop.

o   Don't have unprotected sex
with outsiders.

On the off chance that you figure
you may have any sort of issue
with your liver, or inconveniences
from any condition that you have,

contact your primary care physician.

How might I detox my liver at home?

Garlic: Garlic contains selenium, a mineral that detoxifies the liver. It likewise can actuate liver compounds that can help your body normally flush out poisons. Citrus Fruits: Fruits like grapefruit, oranges, limes and lemons all lift the liver's purifying capacity. What would i be able to drink to detox my liver?

These beverages will purge and detox your liver while you rest

1. Detox beverages to wash down your body.

2. Mint tea.

3. Turmeric tea.

4. Ginger and lemon tea.

5. Fenugreek water.

6. Chamomile tea.

7. Oatmeal and cinnamon drink.

To what extent does it take for your liver to recoup?

The liver, be that as it may, can supplant harmed tissue with new cells. On the off chance that up to 50 to 60 percent of the liver cells might be killed inside three to four days in an outrageous case like a Tylenol overdose, the liver will fix totally following 30 days if no complexities emerge.

What are a portion of the side effects of liver sickness?

The most significant thing to perceive about liver malady is that up to 50 percent of people with basic liver ailment have no manifestations. The most well-known manifestations are very vague and they incorporate weakness or extreme tiredness, absence of drive, and in some cases tingling. Indications of liver sickness that are increasingly conspicuous are jaundice or yellowing of the eyes and skin, dim pee, pale or light shaded stool, seeping from the GI tract, mental disarray, and maintenance of liquids in the mid-region or tummy.

What amount of liquor use ought to be viewed similar to a hazard to the liver?

Any measure of liquor can deliver harm to the liver. In a generally sound individual with no basic liver issues, the general dependable guideline is distinctive for people:

• Men process and can clear liquor more effectively than ladies because of body size, muscle to fat ratio, and certain proteins, so they should constrain to three to four beverages in a day.

•   Women, in light of similar reasons, should restrict to one to two beverages in a day.

Lager and wine are not "more secure" than bourbon or spirits. One drink is characterized as one shot (1 and 1/4 ounces) of bourbon or spirits, one four-ounce glass of wine, or one 12-ounce brew. On the off chance that an individual has a hidden liver condition, for example, hepatitis B or C, or earlier harm from liquor or different ailments, the liver is delicate to any measure of liquor. In those conditions, the main safe portion of liquor is zero.

I realize liquor abuse harms the liver, what other poisonous substances are there those will do harm?

The most widely recognized operator is presumably acetaminophen (Tylenol, in spite of the fact that it is contained in numerous OTC meds). It remains the most secure prescription for fevers, throbs, and torments, yet just taken in little suggested sums. Sums more noteworthy than those suggested can bring about liver harm or disappointment. Acetaminophen overdose is a typical purpose behind thinking about a liver transplant.

A progressively significant issue happens in patients who drink liquor every day, especially multiple beverages. In those circumstances, typical portions of Tylenol three to four times each day can deliver serious liver harm. A similar issue can happen in patients with the other liver maladies, for example, viral hepatitis. Moreover, increasingly regular poisons will in general be those that are breathed in, for example, cleaning solvents, aerosolized paints, thinners, and so on which are progressively perilous with a fundamental condition.

Would liver be able to harm be switched?

The liver is an interesting organ. It is the main organ in the body that can recover. With most organs, for example, the heart, the harmed tissue is supplanted with scar, as on the skin. The liver, be that as it may, can supplant harmed tissue with new cells. On the off chance that up to 50 to 60 percent of the liver cells might be killed inside three to four days in an extraordinary case like a Tylenol overdose, the liver will fix totally following 30 days if no entanglements emerge.

Intricacies of liver ailment happen when recovery is either deficient or averted by dynamic advancement of scar tissue inside the liver. This happens when the harming operator, for example, an infection, a medication, liquor, and so on., keeps on assaulting the liver and forestalls total recovery.

When scar tissue has created it is extremely hard to turn around that procedure. Extreme scarring of the liver is the condition known as cirrhosis. The advancement of cirrhosis shows late stage liver ailment and is typically trailed by the beginning of inconveniences.

To what extent would i be able to continue drinking each prior day it influences my liver?

The biggest hazard factor for liver infection from liquor is the sum and the time span the individual has been drinking. Guys regularly create difficulties that have all the earmarks of being on a sexual orientation premise too. Every individual is altogether extraordinary. Inconvenience can create following 5 to 10 years, however it all the more normally it takes 20 to 30 years. Numerous people appear to never create end arrange liver malady from liquor. This is difficult to foresee early. What's more, numerous different factors, for example, different illnesses, hepatitis C, presentation to different poisons, just as the person's very own hereditary make-up assume a job.

CHAPTER THREE

Citrus natural products

Lemons, tangerines, and oranges contain a compound called D-limonene, which has been appeared to help turn around oxidative harm caused to the liver because of a high-fat eating regimen. Tasting on lemon water for the duration of the day is likewise an incredible method to remain hydrated, which advances the development of poisons out of the body.

Dandelion root and greens

Dandelion is known for its purging properties, and one examination found that both the root and leaf free the collection of receptive oxygen species that reason oxidative pressure. Receive the rewards by tasting on dandelion root tea, which makes an extraordinary without caffeine option in contrast to espresso. Dandelion greens (alongside other harsh greens, for example, mustard greens and arugula) are incredible, as well, as they can help invigorate bile creation and advance sound assimilation.

Aged nourishments

Sauerkraut, kimchi, fermented tea, lacto-aged pickles, kefir, yogurt, and other matured nourishments are stacked with gainful probiotic microscopic organisms that advance solid assimilation and trustworthiness of the gut lining, in this way helping keep poisons out of the circulatory system. As indicated by utilitarian medication master Frank Lipman, M.D., they may likewise help get substantial metals out of the body.

Glutathione-boosting nourishments

Glutathione is a cancer prevention agent gathered stuck the liver that helps spot poisons and escort them out of the body through pee or bile. Glutathione can be gotten straightforwardly from a couple of nourishments, including crude spinach, avocado, and asparagus, and it can likewise be created by your body from the amino acids glutamine, glycine, and cysteine. Nourishments containing the structure squares of glutathione incorporate bone stock, whey protein, and sulfur-containing food sources, for example, broccoli and garlic.

Green tea

Notwithstanding lessening aggravation, phytochemicals in

green tea may help trigger both stage one and stage two liver detoxification. In stage one, poisons are made water-dissolvable by compounds, and in stage two, poisons are bound to defensive synthetic compounds that kill them and enable them to be dispensed with by means of bile or pee.

Verdant greens

Dull verdant greens, for example, dandelion greens, arugula, spinach, and kale contain plant chlorophylls, which help expel synthetic compounds, pesticides, and substantial metals from the circulatory system. In particular, early research shows that chlorophyll may diminish the danger of liver harm brought about by aflatoxins (hazardous mixes delivered by growths that might be available on an assortment of nourishments, including peanuts) by initiating certain chemicals.

Lentils

Get enough fiber-rich nourishments to tie up poisons in the gut and help advance consistency. In case you're obstructed, poisons from the entrail can be reabsorbed into your framework. Attempt vegetables (particularly lentils), raspberries, root vegetables, apples, pears, avocados, and almonds.

Salmon

There are a lot of motivations to get more omega-3 unsaturated fats in your eating routine, and now the wellbeing of your liver is one of them. An ongoing examination survey found that omega-3 utilization was related with lower liver-fat levels and higher HDL "great" cholesterol levels. Other great wellsprings of these solid fats incorporate sardines, pecans, and flaxseed.

Attempt a type of irregular fasting.

A supplement rich diet is critical. In any case, when you've aced that, you might need to consider irregular fasting for extra liver detox support. Research proposes that during times of fasting, cells in the liver produce even more a protein related with improved sugar digestion and diminished degrees of liver fat.

More research around there is required, however various specialists advance irregular fasting for an assortment of reasons. "I love the power that irregular fasting can have on the body's normal detox forms," William Cole, D.C., practical prescription master and smash hit creator of Ketotarian, told mbg. "Periods without nourishment allow our body [and liver] to fix and get itself out since it doesn't need to concentrate on or channel vitality to our stomach related framework.

"Think about this as your body's opportunity to leave work and make up for lost time with some house keeping. One of the cool self-cleaning devices used during fasting is something many refer to as autophagy, which truly means 'self-eating.' When this procedure is permitted to accomplish its thing, our body's sound cells eat up any undesirable cells, prompting a genuine cell detox."

A decent prologue to irregular fasting is the 16-hour quick, where you keep the entirety of your every day eating to an eight-hour window and quick for the rest of the day. Attempt this for possibly 14 days and check whether you see any adjustments in vitality and state of mind. For increasingly explicit direction, look at our complete manual for discontinuous fasting.

CHAPTER FOUR

Do liver rinses work?

Liver rinses guarantee to free the collection of poisons and debasements, yet they are disputable in light of the fact that there is little science to help their utilization.

Items that guarantee to detox the liver may even be hazardous, and the United States Food and Drug Administration (FDA) don't direct them.

In this article, we take a gander at how liver washes down guarantee to function and what proof exists to help them.

What is a liver wash down?

A liver scrub may include may include picking or maintaining a strategic distance from explicit nourishments, or going on a juice quick.

The liver is the body's common detoxifier, as it rinses the assemblage of poisons and creates bile to help solid absorption. A sound liver can detoxify nearly everything that an individual experiences. The liver is on the correct side of the body, simply under the rib confine,

At the point when the liver is unhealthy, the body can't sift through lethal substances as productively. This can cause a wide scope of side effects, including:

- itching

- yellow embittered skin

- swelling

- blood vessel issues

- gallstones

- fatigue

- nausea

- diarrhea

An assortment of common wellbeing specialists, supplement organizations, and medicinal sites contend that the liver collects poisons during the sifting procedure.

They demand that after some time, these poisons can cause a scope of vague side effects and may even reason genuine maladies or increment the danger of malignant growth. There is little proof to help this.

After some time, be that as it may, introduction to synthetic concoctions can harm the liver. For instance, drinking liquor is an outstanding method to destroy liver capacity after some time.

Much of the time, a liver detox includes at least one of the accompanying:

• taking enhancements intended to flush poisons out of the liver

• eating a liver-accommodating eating routine

• avoiding certain nourishments

- going on a juice quick

- cleansing the colon and gut using bowel purges

While liver disappointment is a genuine medical issue, there is no proof that risky poisons collect in generally solid livers without explicit introduction to a lot of these synthetic concoctions.

Standard therapeutic experts contend that the liver doesn't need detoxing and that doing so may even be perilous.

Liver rinse: Fact or fiction?

A liver rinse won't fix a liver sickness, and ought not be utilized to supplant typical treatment.

A solid liver normally washes down itself. An unfortunate liver won't show signs of improvement with a liver purify. An individual with liver sickness needs legitimate therapeutic treatment and may require way of life or dietary changes.

Some proof proposes that enhancements, for example, milk thorn, may improve liver wellbeing. Nonetheless, there is no proof that these enhancements will detox the liver, or that they can fix any liver condition.

Liver washes down additionally represent some wellbeing dangers:

• Liver purging weight control plans may not offer adjusted nourishment: A liver purifying eating routine may not contain all supplements that an individual requires. After some time, this can prompt lacks or hunger, especially in kids, pregnant ladies, and individuals with diabetes and other ailments.

• Enemas can be perilous: Enemas can cause dangerous harm to the digestive organs when not regulated effectively.

• Liver washes down can't supplant restorative treatment: When an individual uses a liver scrub instead of medicinal treatment, genuine fundamental therapeutic issues can go untreated.

Could purging the liver assist you with getting more fit?

Some liver washes down guarantee to help weight reduction by improving an individual's digestion. Supporters accept that flushing the liver of poisons can improve digestion, however there is no proof to help this case.

Actually, extremely low-calorie diets can slow the body's digestion. This is on the grounds that the body changes with the low supplement consumption by retaining supplements all the more gradually.

A few eats less that guarantee to improve liver wellbeing expect individuals to expend not many calories for a few days. This can bring about transitory weight reduction.

A significant part of the weight reduction, be that as it may, is water weight, which will return once an individual starts to eat typically once more.

THE END

www.ingramcontent.com/pod-product-compliance
Lightning Source LLC
Chambersburg PA
CBHW070516220526
45467CB00002B/701

* 9 7 8 1 7 0 4 8 2 2 3 2 7 *